The Gallstone Diet

Foods for Your Gallbladder

Prevent, Manage, and Flush your Gallstones

By

Anna Keating

The Gallstone Diet: Foods for Your Gallbladder - Prevent, Manage, and Flush your Gallstones

ISBN-10: 1549760068

ISBN-13: 978-1549760068

Warning and Disclaimer

Every effort has been made to make this book as accurate as possible. However, no warranty or fitness is implied. The information provided is on an "as-is" basis. The author and the publisher shall have no liability or responsibility to any person or entity with respect to any loss or damages that arise from the information in this book.

Publisher contact

Skinny Bottle Publishing

books@skinnybottle.com

About the author

After having a near-death experience due to an organ failure, Anna Keating promised that she would take a better care of herself. Twenty years later, she is a mother of three healthy children and a health advocate who helps others avoid the complications she went through.

Sharing her knowledge and experience with the rest of the world, Anna has a lot to say about our overall health. If you want to avoid health complications due to an unhealthy lifestyle and imbalanced diet, then you have come to the right place.

ANNA KEATING

The Only "Medication"

Just because you have been diagnosed with gallstones in your gallbladder doesn't mean that you are about to spend the rest of your life in pain and agony, or undergo a surgical procedure by default.

If one thing is certain, it is that once they are formed, gallstones are there to stay. If you want to keep your gallbladder and spare yourself some severely painful gallstone attacks, I suggest you learn how to live with those lumps inside your gallbladder.

The best, well actually, the only "medication" that has been proven to keep gallstone symptoms at bay, is a properly balanced diet. Whether your gallstones show no symptoms, you have suffered a couple of painful gallstone episodes, or have unfortunately lost your gallbladder due to these annoying pebbles, one thing is certain, this book will help you live a hale and hearty life.

From why and how they are developed, through all of the treatment options available, this book provides you with the knowledge to understand why a proper gallstone diet is of great importance. Introducing to you the ultimate gallstone diet and getting you started with a ridiculously delicious 6-week gallstone diet meal plan, this book will be your best friend during this not so fun journey.

Together we can win the fight that you may think is over.

Inside the Gallbladder

We usually don't even give the gallbladder a thought. Unlike the liver or the kidneys, this small, pear-shaped pouch is often neglected. Maybe it's because we know that the gallbladder isn't exactly crucial for the proper functioning of our body. Maybe it's the fact that we don't hear enough about gallbladder health, I'm not sure. But what I do know is that even though it may not be one of the most important organs in our body, the gallbladder has indeed an important job.

The gallbladder is a small organ that is tucked below the right rib cage, just under the liver. Its size varies from person to person and can be as small as a plum, or as big as a large apple. It is actually attached to the liver, resting on top of the small bowel. The gallbladder is connected to the intestines with small tubes that are called bile ducts. These bile ducts are in charge of carrying the yellow/greenish fluid (bile) that is produced by the liver.

So what exactly is bile and why is it important? Like I said, bile is a fluid produced by the liver and stored in the gallbladder that helps with digestion. Bile supports proper absorption of fats, as well as other fat-soluble substances (think vitamins A, D, E, and K). Bile contains water, phospholipids and cholesterol, as well as other chemicals that support digestion. But besides promoting proper digestion, bile is also important to our body because it is an important excretion 'route' for many waste products, such as bilirubin (the red blood cells' byproduct that is recycled by the liver).

The gallbladder expands when bile accumulates and this mostly happens when a person hasn't eaten in a long time period; for instance, if the person is sick, fasting, or is dieting severely and follows a fad diet. The main job of the gallbladder is to collect and store the bile, and then release it during food consumption into the bile ducts. The bile is then transferred via the ducts to our intestine. There, the bile breaks up the consumed fat into tiny droplets that can be easily absorbed. Now, since the bile is stored in the gallbladder, the importance of the gallbladder is pretty obvious.

It all sounds pretty normal, so how are gallstones developed? When does this disruption occur? To understand how gallstones are formed, experts suggest picturing the organs for digestion as a 'biliary tree'. This biliary tree involves four organs that are connected to each other with tubes. To understand this even better, just picture yourself drawing a diagram that features your liver, gallbladder, pancreas, and small bowel. The liver is on the top of the diagram, the gallbladder is on the right, pancreas on the left, and finally the small bowel at the bottom. All of these organs are connected to each other with crisscrossed pipes. Does it get clearer?

The point of this biliary tree is to transfer the secretions throughout this body which will at the same time support digestion, absorb nutrients, and eliminate waste. The cycle starts with the liver, of course, then the secretions move to the gallbladder, then go in and out of the pancreas and end up in the small bowel. The purpose of this cycle is to purge the waste out of the body in the form of a yellow/greenish fluid called bile.

What you perhaps don't know, is the fact that the body does not get rid of bile constantly. Instead, it stores bile and similar secretion and uses them when they are needed. The body decides to hold on to bile so it can be used efficiently and immediately when we begin to eat, in order to support proper digestion.

The bile duct, which is basically a muscle that resembles a valve, is closed when there is no food in the small bowel and gets opened up once we start ingesting food, so that bile, secretions and other important enzymes can pass through and contribute to normal digestion.

And while the bile ducts get closed when there is no more food in the small bowel (for example, when fasting), the liver and pancreas have no way of knowing this so they do not close the doors and stop working. They constantly produce secretions, as well as bile. And since they are also unaware of our eating schedule, or whether we have an appetite or not, they receive absolutely no sign that they should stop production. That is why digestive secretions, bile included, are pumped out constantly, meaning that there is always extra bile inside. But what happens when the bile ducts receive the message that there is no need for bile in the small bowel and close themselves up, and the liver and pancreas don't? Where does the bile go in that case? When the bile is released from the gallbladder and reaches a closed bile duct, it has no choice but to return inside the gallbladder.

So back to the importance of the gallbladder. This pear-shaped organ is important for digestion because it collects the extra bile that cannot be transferred to the small bowel, and stores it in a safe place. Once we start eating, the gallbladder will contract itself, which will squeeze out the bile that contributes to smooth digestion.

So, how is this cycle disrupted? Actually, not every doctor and specialist agrees upon the exact reason for developing gallstones. However, one of the main theories is that when the cholesterol from the bile binds with some of the other bile matter, it becomes more solid and gets lodged in the gallbladder's inner lining. Over time, this cholesterol that gets stuck to the gallbladder's wall grows and forms stone-like solid particles known as gallstones.

Gallstones Under the Spotlight

Gallstones, as the name suggests, are solid particles that look like stones and are formed inside the gallbladder. Gallstones, or as doctors like to call them cholelithiasis, are made up of particles of cholesterol, calcium deposits, and some other substances that can be found in bile. Their shape and size, as well as density and composition vary from person to person, but all gallstones are caused and treated the same way.

They can be as tiny as a sand grain or as large as a golf ball. However, even though they are called 'stone' these lumps of solid material are not that solid. Since they are mostly made of cholesterol, which is not solid, the gallstones are not rock hard and compared to kidney stones, they are much softer.

The composition of the gallstones mainly depends on the age of the person, the diet they consume, or even their ethnicity. Based on their composition, gallstones can be divided into three types:

Cholesterol Stones – Cholesterol stones are the most common type of gallstones that people suffer from. As I explained earlier, they are formed due to the binding of cholesterol with other bile matter after which they form more solid lumps that get stuck to the gallbladder wall. They can be yellow, dark green, brown, or even chalk white in color. The shape is mostly oval and they have a dark spot in the center.

Bilirubin Stones – Bilirubin stones are primarily made of bilirubin, as well as calcium salts that can be found in bile. Bilirubin stones are small, usually numerous, and have a dark, almost black color.

7

Brown Pigment Stones – Brown pigment, also called mixed stones contain about 20 to 80 percent cholesterol as well as calcium carbonate, bilirubin, palmitate phosphate, and other bile substances. Due to their calcium content, these stones are almost always radiographically visible.

The Cause

Like I said, it is somewhat unclear what exactly causes gallstones to develop in the gallbladder, but these are the theories that have been accepted by doctors:

Too much cholesterol

Eating a food high in fat and high in cholesterol will eventually cause the cholesterol to pile up in your bile. This, of course, doesn't happen by default, but it is known that if your bile contains too much cholesterol, you will most likely have cholesterol gallstones developinside your gallbladder.

Too much bilirubin

When your body gets rid of old and unused red blood cells, a chemical called bilirubin is produced. If your liver produces more bilirubin than it should, which sometimes happens as a result of some blood disorders or liver damage, you are at risk for developing bilirubin or pigment gallstones. When there is excess bilirubin that the gallbladder cannot efficiently break down, dark bilirubin stones are formed inside.

Concentrated Bile

To be able to function properly the gallbladder needs to be empty. If the gallbladder, for some reason, fails to get rid of the excess bile that is stored inside, the bile will get over concentrated, which will lead to the development of gallstones.

Risk Factors

Who is most likely to develop gallstones? There are many factors that can contribute to the formation of gallstones including the diet that people consume, their age, sex, genetics and body composition.

Gallstones are most common among:

-   Women

-   People over 40

-   Overweight and obese people

Some of the common factors also include:

-   Pregnancy

-   Diabetes

-   Sedentary lifestyle

-   Losing weight quickly (for instance, after fasting)

-   Family history of gallstones

-   Low HDL cholesterol

-   Consuming an imbalanced diet

- High triglyceride levels

- Liver disease

- Medications with estrogen, contraceptive drugs or hormone therapy drugs

You must be wondering why this is the case. The thing that contributes to the development of gallstones the most is hormonal imbalances. That is the reason why women are more likely to develop gallstones than men. And that is especially the case with those women that are either pregnant or are on birth control pills. Experts believe it is the female sex hormone called estrogen that is mostly to blame.

Estrogen is known to have the ability to increase the cholesterol in the bile, as well as to decrease the proper functioning of the bladder (meaning to decrease its contractions), both of which can contribute to the creation of gallstones in the gallbladder.

Another thing you should know, which may confuse some of you, is that taking drugs that help you lower cholesterol levels can actually cause cholesterol gallstones. These drugs may lower the cholesterol levels in your blood, but they may increase the cholesterol in the bile, which may set the scene for the cholesterol gallstones to appear in the gallbladder.

How to Detect Them?

The thing about gallstones is that they don't usually let you know that they are there until it is too late. That is why they are often called 'silent stones', since most of them show no symptoms at all. In fact, most people with gallstones are not even aware of these lumps in their gallbladder. The majority of gallstones are detected by accident, whether during an abdominal ultrasound, stomach surgery, or some other physical examination.

However, some gallstones cause severe pain. The symptoms, of course, vary from person to person, but usually, when a person is experiencing a 'gallstone attack' they are going through a lot of pain. Usually, these attacks happen at night.

The symptoms also depend on the location of the gallstone. And while all gallstones are born in the gallbladder, they can easily get dislocated and move to different parts such as the bile duct. Sometimes, they might even end up in the small bowel.

The most painful attacks happen as a result of the blockage that gallstones can make in the bile ducts. Sometimes, a gallstone can be moved to the bile duct and block the valve completely, and with that also block the bile's path to the small bowel. When this happens and the gallbladder contracts, squeezing the bile out, the bile has nowhere to go, which can cause severe pain. This is known as biliary colic.

These are the symptoms that someone with a gallstone may experience:

-        Sudden and severe pain in the abdomen that can last from 30 minutes to several hours.

-        The pain usually starts under the ribs on the right side, and it may easily spread to the shoulder blade or side. The pain can also be felt in the center of the tummy.

-        Tension in the intestines after meals.

Know that the pain that happens as a result of a gallstone is constant. That means that it does not subside or go away if you change positions or go to the toilet.

The tricky part about biliary colic is that it doesn't happen often. You may think that this is a good thing, but many people have let their gallstones cause further complications just because of this. After a gallstone episode is over, it may be months before you experience another. Make sure to contact your doctor immediately after the occurrence of such an episode.

11

I know what you must be thinking; If most of the time gallstones don't show any signs or symptoms, how do you know if you have such a lump in your gallbladder? Like I said, gallstones are usually found by accident, mostly during an abdominal ultrasound for another problem, or during pregnancy. But, if you want to have your gallbladder checked for gallstones, you can surely contact your doctor and get yourself tested. And while a physical exam or your medical history may indicate that you have gallstones, your doctor will perform some of the following tests to confirm:

Abdominal Ultrasound – This is the most common, the simplest, and probably the best test for diagnosing gallstones. The abdominal ultrasound is performed with a wand that a technician moves around the belly in order to show pictures of your organs on a video monitor. Usually, this is the only test that is needed for diagnosing gallstones.

Gallbladder Scan – Even if your abdominal ultrasound shows no signs of gallstones, your doctor may still think that you have a lump inside your gallbladder due to some other signs or risks that may suggest that. When that is the case, doctors usually suggest gallbladder scan. The gallbladder scan is performed after the doctor injects a radioactive dye into a vein in one of the arms in order to take pictures and see if the gallbladder is functioning properly. This scan may also show other problems like blocked bile ducts.

ERCP (Endoscopic Retrograde Cholangiopancreatogram) – This test is performed to see if there is a gallstone inside the bile ducts that connect your liver with the gallbladder, pancreas or small bowel. The ERCP is done after the doctor inserts and moves a light and very flexible instrument down your throat in order to check those tubes that drain the gallbladder, liver, and pancreas.

Blood Test – A complete blood test, including tests for pancreatitis and liver function, may indicate abnormal liver function. These tests are great because if there isn't a gallstone that has been causing you a severe pain, they will most likely reveal the cause of your problems.

Endoscopic Ultrasound (EUS) – Similar to the ERCP, the endoscopic ultrasound is also a test that involves a lightweight and flexible instrument to be moved down your throat and into your stomach in order for the tubes that drain your digestive organs to be examined. The only difference between these two similar procedures is that the ERCP uses a camera in order to generate a video image, while the EUS is an ultrasound, meaning that it shows images with high-frequency sound waves.

Magnetic Resonance Cholangiogram (MRC) – This is a test that uses MRI or magnetic field and radio wave energy pulses in order to provide images of the organs and structures inside the abdomen. This is usually the test that doctors perform before removing the gallbladder or in order to detect some other gallbladder and bile duct problems.

Complications

Most people that have gallstones never even experience symptoms, let alone have complications. But while complications caused by stones in the gallbladder are indeed rare, gallstones can still cause:

Cholecystitis

Cholecystitis is an inflammation of the gallbladder that is usually caused when there is a gallstone located in the gallbladder's neck or the cystic duct (which is one of the bile ducts). Cholecystitis is usually triggered after consuming a large, fatty meal.

The symptoms of cholecystitis are:

- Severe pain in the upper part of the abdomen that usually lasts for more than 12 hours.

- Tenderness in the abdomen

- Vomiting and nausea

13

-     Fever

The cholecystitis symptoms are different than those when there is biliary colic present. The pain here is sharper, lasts longer, and is followed by a fever, which does not occur during biliary colic. Also, when there is biliary colic, the abdomen does not feel overly tender when touched.

Cholangitis

While cholecystitis is an inflammation of the gallbladder, cholangitis is an inflammation of the bile ducts. This usually occurs after the ducts become blocked and then infected by some bacteria from the small bowel. The symptoms include:

-     Fever

-     Abdominal pain

-     Jaundice – yellow discoloration of the whites of the eyes as well as the skin.

If you experience these symptoms make sure to visit the nearest hospital since cholangitis is a serious condition that requires urgent treatment.

Acute Biliary Pancreatitis

Pancreatitis is an inflammation of the pancreas and it is a serious disorder that sometimes occurs when there is a gallstone present. Pancreatitis happens when there is a gallstone blocking the pancreatic duct (which is the bile duct leading from the pancreas), and usually, this disorder occurs when there are numerous gallstones present.

The symptoms include:

- Nausea and vomiting

- Severe pain in the upper part of the abdomen that goes through the back

- Fever

Gallstone Ileus

When there is a gallstone obstructing the large or small intestine, gallstone ileus may occur. This is a condition that usually happens when a gallbladder that has been previously inflamed gets stuck to the intestine. When this happens, the gallstones can go through the wall of the gallbladder and into the intestine, causing a blockage. The symptoms include:

- Abdominal pain

- Bloating of the abdomen

- Nausea and Vomiting

- Constipation

Gallbladder Cancer

Although this is extremely rare, having gallstones in the gallbladder does increase the risk for gallbladder cancer.

Treating Gallstones

The treatment of the gallstones depends on the person's unique condition as well as the stage of the disease, but mostly, the treatment plan for gallstones mainly depends on how the disease affects the person's daily life.

If you have been diagnosed with a gallstone and want to know your treatment options, then this chapter will present to with all of your options. Just remember that the complications that may happen as a result of a gallstone also depend on your overall health, so, if your doctor believes it is best for you to undergo a certain treatment, you should give it serious thought.

Asymptomatic Gallstones

Those gallstones that are present in the gallbladder but show no signs or symptoms of their presence are called asymptomatic gallstones. And while it may seem scary to have a solid lump in your gallbladder, most asymptomatic gallstones do not require any special treatment, except healthy management.

People with asymptomatic gallstones are not encouraged not to remove them surgically. In fact, the risk that may arise after such an intervention is actually greater than the risk that the gallstones will cause complications. On average, only 25 percent of people who have asymptomatic gallstones will develop symptoms in the next ten years.

The 'rule' is that if your gallstones are not telling you that they are there – do not wake them up. It has been proven that the longer people with asymptomatic gallstones go without symptoms, the less likely it is that their gallbladder disease will get worse.

However, not all people with asymptomatic gallstones are encouraged not to treat them. Here is why your doctor may suggest an immediate treatment even if your gallstones are asymptomatic:

-        The gallstones are larger than 2 or 3 cm in diameter. If the stone in your gallbladder is pretty large, your doctor may suggest certain treatments in order to stop further complications that are most likely to happen in such cases.

-        You have scarring of the liver, known as cirrhosis.

-        You have high blood pressure inside the liver, known as portal hypertension (this usually happens because of cirrhosis).

-        You have diabetes. Depending on the severity and type of your diabetes, your doctor may suggest gallstone treatment if he or she thinks that this lump in your gallbladder with the combination of your blood sugar disease may cause your health some serious complications.

-        There are high levels of calcium in the gallbladder. High levels of calcium in the gallbladder are the main indicator that you are a good candidate for developing a gallbladder cancer later in life. If that is the case with you, your doctor may suggest a more invasive treatment.

-        You have sickle cell anemia and it is difficult for your doctor to distinguish what are painful crises due to that disease and what may be cholecystitis.

-        You have a spinal cord injury that may affect your abdomen.

People with asymptomatic gallstones are mostly encouraged not to seek any special treatment but manage their condition by being active and following a special gallstone diet (which this book provides) in order to prevent the symptoms from occurring and stop the formation of new gallstones. However, if you are frightened by the small risk of developing a gallbladder cancer or you simply think that getting rid of the gallstone or gallbladder is a better option for you then you should definitely present your worries to your doctor, with whom you can discuss your options and find the best treatment for your unique condition. The next section covers all of the treatment options available.

Symptomatic Gallstones

When gallstones begin showing symptoms, it is a sign that they should definitely be treated. However, not all people who have symptomatic gallstones will end up on the operating table. Depending on the person's condition and the severity of this gallbladder disease there are a couple of surgical and non-surgical interventions that may treat the patient.

Medical Dissolution

If the condition is not that severe and you are not a surgery candidate but your gallstones are still interfering with your normal life, your doctor might suggest medical dissolution. Even if you have no symptoms you may ask your doctor to try this option.

For this treatment, doctors usually prescribe ursodiol which is ursodeoxycholic acid. Ursodiol is a dissolution agent that can sometimes help in dissolving gallstones. The long-term administration of ursodiol may reduce the concentration of the cholesterol in the bile by reducing the detergent effect that the gallbladder's bile salts have, as well as reducing the liver's secretion of cholesterol.

A treatment of 8 to 10 mg (per kg per day) of ursodeoxycholic acid tablets for 6 to 18 months may contribute to a gradual dissolution of the gallstones, however, this is successful only for really small, and only cholesterol, gallstones.

Despite their ability to help with dissolution, the ursodiol is rarely prescribed because:

- It is rarely effective

- The patients need to take the tablets for a long time

- Once the treatment is stopped, gallstones have a 50 percent chance of recurring within 5 years.

Surgical Removal

It is estimated that every year, in North America alone, there are over 750,000 gallbladder surgeries performed due to painful gallstones. If the patient has severe abdominal pain, gallbladder inflammation, or falls into one of the previously mentioned groups of people that can suffer further complications due to gallstones, a surgery is performed.

Unfortunately, when we say surgery they do not simply removethe gallstones, but the whole gallbladder. And while it is an important digestive organ, the gallbladder isn't exactly essential for living a healthy and normal life.

There are two ways in which the gallbladder can be removed:

Keyhole Surgery or Laparoscopic Cholecystectomy

Usually, when doctors suggest a surgical gallbladder removal they mean laparoscopic cholecystectomy. This surgery is performed with three or four small abdominal cuts: the largest one is approximately 2-3 cm long and it is by the belly button, and the other two which are 1 cm long or less, are on the right side of the abdomen.

During this procedure, the abdomen is inflated with carbon dioxide gas, which enables the doctor to fully see the abdominal organs and perform the operation successfully.

Then, a laparoscope, a small tube that has a camera attached to it, is inserted through one of the abdominal cuts. This allows the doctor to watch the operation on a monitor. The gallbladder is removed with special instruments. If there are gallstones in the bile ducts as well, they can also be removed during this keyhole surgery.

After the gallbladder has been removed, the abdominal gas escapes through the tube of the laparoscope, and the cuts are closed, usually with dissolvable stitches. The operation doesn't takes60 – 90 minutes, it is performed under general anesthesia, and you get to go home the same day. The full recovery takes about 10 days.

Open Surgery

Before keyhole surgery, the traditional way of removing the gallbladder was with open surgery. Open surgery is not less effective than the keyhole surgery, they're pretty much equally successful at safely removing the gallbladder. The only thing that makes this surgery less appealing is the fact that instead of three small cuts the surgeon makes one large abdominal incision (10-15 cm long) just under the ribcage in order to remove the gallbladder. Besides the large and visible scarring, the open surgery also requires a hospital day of at least 5 days and full recovery usually takes 6 weeks.

Many people, however, are still candidates for an open surgery:

- Women that are in their third trimester

- People that are extremely overweight

- People who have an unusual gallbladder or whose bile duct structure makes it impossible for the surgeons to perform a successful keyhole surgery

ERCP

Endoscopic Retrograde Cholangio Pancreatography isn't only performed in order to detect gallstones, but also to remove them. This procedure is performed only for the removal of those gallstones that are in the bile duct. If you have a gallstone that has moved to the bile duct, chances are, it can be removed directly from the bile duct without removing the gallbladder. However, if you have other gallstones in the gallbladder they cannot be removed unless you undergo a surgical procedure.

The ERCP, as I said before, is performed when the doctor inserts an endoscope down your throat, all the way to where the bile ducts open into the small bowel. In order to remove the gallstone, the bile duct is widened with a small incision or with a heated wire. Then the stones can be either removed or left to pass through the small bowel and out of the body.

In some cases, the doctors place stents in the bile duct, which are small tubes that can 'grease' the path and help the bile and gallstones pass freely.

The patient is sedated, but awake during this procedure, and the ERCP lasts for about half an hour on average.

Lithotripsy

Lithotripsy, also called shock wave therapy, is a procedure that uses ultrasound waves in order to break up gallstones. Although it can be used alone, this therapy is often used along with bile acids so the chances of breakup and dissolution are increased. These ultrasound waves break up the gallstones into tiny pieces that are easier to dissolve. That is why the bile acid tablets are encouraged to speed up the process.

However painless and efficient this may seem, know that the lithotripsy is not performed that often. It is used only for stones that are smaller than 2 cm, and mostly for people who are either unwilling or cannot undergo a surgical procedure.

The shock wave therapy is not appropriate for treating severe and acute cholecystitis.

Healthifying Your Diet

If there has been a gallstone detected in your gallbladder, don't worry. That does not mean that you have to remove your gallbladder or experience further complications that may interfere with your normal life. Quite the contrary, actually. Many gallstones almost never cause complications. However, in order for you to minimalize the risk that gallstones are known to carry to some extent, as well as to prevent the cholesterol from piling up inside your gallbladder and stop new gallstones from forming, it is of great importance that you make some great lifestyle changes.

Since the gallbladder is a digestive organ, it is pretty clear how an improper and imbalanced diet can contribute to its disease. That being said, one of the most important, if not the most crucial, things you can do in order to manage the gallstones and prevent them from causing further health problems is to change your unhealthy diet.

I know that living with gallstones may not feel like the best option, but know that if you do not fall under the risk group and your doctor has assured you that it is riskier to treat than it is to learn to live with the gallstone, a healthy and proper gallstone diet is all it will take for you to reach your senior years hale and hearty.

But, before we dive into what should be put on your plate, let us make some room for the healthy ingredients first. Now, roll up your sleeves because we are about to makeover and healthify your kitchen completely. Here is what shouldn't be included in your diet when you have gallstones:

Processed Food

I guess this doesn't really need an explanation since we all know that a well-balanced diet should be free of processed food. However, processed foods shouldn't only be banned because they are filled with unhealthy and fattening ingredients that will make the numbers on the scale skyrocket. When it comes to gallstones, the main reason why you should purge processed food out of your diet is the fact that it is packed with chemicals that 'mimic' the effects of estrogen, which contributes to creating excess estrogen that can slow down the breakdown of fat cells.

Sugar

Of course, sugar isn't allowed. This sweet hazard is not only to blame for the fact that you can no longer fit in your old jeans, but it is also the cause of many other health issues. Forming gallstones is one of them. To simplify things; sugar leads to gaining weight and inflammation which increases the risk of developing gallstones significantly.

Fatty Meat

You don't have to go full vegetarian in order to avoid the fat from the meat. Meat is a healthy protein source and is therefore extremely important for proper body function. However, you have to be careful about the type of meat that you consume. Meat with fatty content such as sausages, lunch meat, and pork should not be a part of a healthy gallstone diet. Now, when it comes to red meat, it is best to limit it to one or maybe two portions a week, and choose only the leanest cuts. Always go for the organic, grass-fed only meat.

When cooking poultry, make sure to use only skinless meat to avoid gallstone irritation.

Fried Food

Deep fried food must be eliminated from your diet if you want to manage your gallstones and keep them asymptomatic. Cooking oils that are high in saturated fat (this also includes foods with saturated fat in general) such as vegetable shortening, animal fat, or margarine, should not be included in your diet. Frying your food with fat that has been partially hydrogenated and contains trans fats and saturated fats will aggravate the gallstone pain and cause discomfort.

Dairy

Experts warn that whole-fat dairy is one of the main reasons for developing gallstone associated complications. The fat content of the dairy poses risks for your gallbladder. It is proinflammatory and it will not only contribute to further complications like severe pain and discomfort, but it will also help new gallstones form. That is why it is of crucial importance not to use whole-fat milk and conventional milk products like cheese, ice cream and frozen yogurt..

Refined Foods

If you have been diagnosed with gallstones, then you should definitely refrain from eating refined food. Refined ingredients found in white bread, white rice, white pasta, etc., get easily converted to stored fat during the digestion process, which can increase the cholesterol levels in the bile and make your gallstones grow, as well as contribute to the formation of new stones.

Eggs

If you have been diagnosed and have spent some time online reading about the best diet to follow, then you must have come across the theory that eggs should be eliminated from the healthy gallstone diet. I just want to make something very clear before you accept everything that is written online. Eggs are extremely healthy. Yes, they may have higher cholesterol levels, but all of their other healthy properties diminish that. Eggs should not be eliminated from your diet. However, do not overindulge. It is okay to have an egg or two occasionally, but don't make eggs the bulk of your every breakfast. Instead, eat eggs in moderation. Eggs are also known to be allergens which can increase the risk of causing gallbladder irritations, but if you are not allergic to them, I don't see why you cannot have a hardboiled egg from time to time.

Gallstone Diet Guidelines

There isn't really a one-of-a-kind diet that can magically help every person that has been diagnosed with gallstones. Some ingredients may help one person, while the same food may cause gallbladder discomfort for others. There isn't really one solution that will fix everyone's gallstone problems. If you were looking for the magical cure, I cannot help you find it. Your unique condition, as well the severity of your gallbladder disease can dictate which ingredients should and shouldn't be put on your table.

However, if you are looking for some general guidelines that have helped the majority of people with gallstones to stop their growth, as well as the occurrence of the new lumps while keeping the symptoms at bay, then this chapter will offer you just that.

The gallstone diet is a combination of the anti-inflammatory and low-fat diet. It is rich in alkaline and anti-inflammatory foods that will purge the toxins out of your body, keeping your organs healthy and free of irritations   This diet is also low in unhealthy fats that may raise your cholesterol and contribute to the growth of the cholesterol lumps in your gallbladder. To make sure your gallbladder will stay safe, follow these guidelines.

The Gallstone Grocery List

Gallstones cannot be cured, and they can rarely be dissolved naturally. However, despite the fact that they take residence in your gallbladder, you two can get along just fine. Think of it this way. If you feed the gallstones what they want to eat, they will not hurt you. Most gallstones never show symptoms. To make sure that it will stay that way, you have to follow a healthy and balanced diet that will not only keep your gallbladder from getting irritated, but will also be beneficial for the rest of your body.

So, forget the aisles where the chips and chocolate hide, and fill your shopping cart with some of these ingredients:

Healthy and Unrefined Fats

Including healthy fats such as olive oil and coconut oil in your diet can really make all the difference for you gallbladder's health. Coconut oil probably contains the most digestible healthy fats called medium-chained fatty acids. Olive oil, especially extra virgin olive oil is packed with anti-inflammatory properties that can help your gallstones pass, and in some cases even dissolve. That's the reason why in the countries where olive oil is mostly consumed, such as the Mediterranean, there are significantly less registered patients with gallstones.

I strongly recommend consuming these healthy fats a couple of times a day, but in small amounts (a tablespoon or so). That way you will make sure that you will not increase your fat intake more than you should, and will put less stress on your gallbladder and liver.

High-Fiber Foods

Fiber is an extremely important macronutrient that is known to support digestion, which at this point, your body really needs. Make sure to incorporate from 30 to 40 grams of fiber every day. This will not only prevent new gallstones from forming, but it will also stop the ones you already have from growing and causing pain. Nuts, beans, and legumes are all welcome.

Many people think that eating these may cause gasses and increase irritation in the gallbladder, but that is not the truth. If you prepare them the right way by soaking your beans and legumes and sprouting your nuts and seeds, your body will digest them easily and you will still get all of the key nutrients.

Whole-Grains

There is no healthy diet that lacks whole grains, so make sure your gallstone diet doesn't either. Whole grains are packed with fiber that prevents the formation of the gallstones. Fiber is known to have the ability to bind together with the cholesterol and bile, and speed up the process of their removal.

Raw Fruits and Vegetables

Raw fruits and vegetables are naturally rich in antioxidants, high in water, and electrolytes, but low in unhealthy fats and salts, which means that they should be the center of your gallstone diet. No, I am not saying that you should go full vegetarian, however, know that increasing the intake of raw and plant-based ingredients is the key to enabling your gallbladder to function properly despite its gallstones.

Make sure to choose antioxidant-rich ingredients that have detoxifying effects and that will support the health of your liver and help the fat cells break down faster, such as artichokes, beets, dandelion leaves, etc.

Also, potassium-rich foods should be on your plate as well. Avocados, dark leafy greens, bananas, sweet potatoes, tomatoes, etc., are both yummy and great for managing gallstones.

Lean Protein Foods

Including protein in your diet is important, but when you have gallstones and you want to keep the symptoms and the pain at bay, it is important to pay attention to the kind of protein you will consume. The safest option for people with gallstones is to choose lean protein sources that are also organic. That includes skinless chicken, turkey, wild-caught fish, organic protein powder, lean red meat in moderation, etc.

Fish and seafood are a healthy addition to the gallstone diet, but you have to be careful. Shellfish like lobster, shrimp, crab, scallops, etc., are really low in fat and excellent for people with gallstones. If your gallstones are symptomatic, limit or avoid the consumption of fatty fish such as salmon, tuna, and trout, and consume only low-fat fish like haddock, cod, pollock, flounder, orange roughy, etc. If you have asymptomatic gallstones, fatty fish is okay to consume from time to time.

No Fat, No Pain!

A diet that is high in fat can even cause discomfort to a healthy person. Now imagine how brutal it will be to a person who suffers from a digestive organ disease. A person whose gallbladder has gallstones and cannot function the way it should. A high-fat diet will not only cause discomfort but may also cause severe pain and force the patients to have their gallbladders removed.

To avoid all that and to enable your gallbladder to function as normal as it should despite the presence of the gallstones, you need to lower the fat intake and reduce the fat cells that should be broken down by your digestive organs.

Note that this will not cure your gallbladder, but support proper functioning and prevent gallstone attacks and acute pain.

And since I know that changing your old habits is easier said than done, I have gathered some general tips that may help you cut down on fat:

-       Cook your meals from scratch. That is the only way of knowing exactly what and how much your meals contain. This will give you control over fat consumption and give you a pretty accurate picture of how much you consume.

-       Always check labels before buying. Look for food that has low fat, not reduced fat. Reduced fat may mean that the fat content is 20 percent reduced, but that doesn't mean that the product is no longer fatty.

-       Cut back on red milk For instance, if you are making spaghetti Bolognese, you can use half of the amount of milk, and add some pureed beans in the sauce, instead.

-       Do not pour oil when cooking, but measure. The rule of thumb is that you should use about 1 teaspoon of fat or oil per person.

-       Buy a cooking spray, or simply pour some olive oil into a clean spray bottle. This will make you use as little oil as possible when cooking.

-       When meat gets stuck to the bottom of the pan, do not add more oil. A drop or two of water will help you scrape the burnt pieces up, without upping the fat content.

-       Remove all visible skin and fat from meat before cooking.

-       When making stews or casseroles, make sure to skim the fat off of the top.

-       Do not fry your food. Bake, boil, grill, steam, or roast instead.

-       Make your own low-fat dressings by using fresh herbs, lemon juice and low-fat yogurt instead of mayonnaise.

Healthier Swaps

If you think that you will have to say goodbye to your favorite food just because you should cut back on fat, then think again. I present to you the ultimate low-fat food swap list that will be much friendlier to your gallbladder and will keep the stones from multiplying, growing, or making further complications.

Butter and ghee - - > Coconut oil

Vegetable Oils - - > Olive oil

Whole-Fat Dairy - - > Low-Fat, Skim, or dairy-free options such as coconut milk, almond milk, coconut cream, etc.

Full-Fat Cheese like Cheddar or Brie - - > Light and soft cheeses such as low-fat cream cheese, cottage cheese, etc.

Puddings and ice cream - - > Frozen Yogurt made with skim yogurt with fresh fruits and no sugar, rice pudding made with skim milk, sorbet, etc.

Cakes, pastries, and biscuits - - > Dried fruit, rice cakes, toasted teacakes, meringues, etc.

Chips and crisps - - > Low-fat popcorn, fruits, and veggies, low-fat crisps

Dresses and sauces - - > Vinaigrette, mustard, lemon juice, low-fat mayonnaise, low-fat yogurt, salsa, balsamic dressing, tomato sauces.

Gallbladder Flush – Natural Remedy or Myth?

A gallbladder flush or gallbladder cleanse is a holistic and natural approach to getting rid of the gallstones from your body with the help of oils, herbs, and juices over the course of a couple days. In most cases, people with gallstones are advised not to eat anything for a long time period during these cleanses or flushes.

There are many recipes and there really isn't one magical formula that can help you get rid of your gallstone, however, different practitioners have different recipes that they follow. The main purpose of this gallbladder flush is for the gallbladder to break up the gallstones gradually, and then release them in the stool.

Many people have said that they have gotten rid of their gallstones this way, however, there is no scientific evidence that can actually support whether this gallbladder flush actually helps people eliminate gallstones in the stool. Besides, fasting for a long time period can never be healthy. For those reasons, I am against the classic gallbladder cleanse.

However, we cannot simply close our eyes to the fact that there are many natural ingredients that are packed with amazing cleansing, anti-inflammatory and digestion-supportive properties that our gallbladder can surely benefit from. And while I cannot really vouch for these natural remedies below and tell you that they will help you dissolve or get rid of your gallstone, they will surely prevent the risks associated with these cholesterol pebbles, stop the acute pain from occurring and make sure they stay asymptomatic. Isn't that what managing the gallstones is all about?

Apple Cider Vinegar

The acidity of the apple cider vinegar stops the liver from making cholesterol, which is the top cause of developing gallstones in the gallbladder. That being said, this magical ingredient is pretty beneficial for your gallbladder disease. If you have gallstone attacks, simply mix one tablespoon of apple cider vinegar in a glass of apple juice. This is supposed to lower the pain within 15 minutes.

If you have asymptomatic gallstones you can mix two teaspoons of apple cider vinegar and one teaspoon of lemon juice in a glass of warm water and drink this solution on an empty stomach, every morning.

Lemon Juice

The pectin found in lemons is known to help in eliminating gallbladder pain that is associated with gallstones. Besides that, the lemon juice also stops the liver from making cholesterol, its vitamin C also makes the cholesterol much more soluble, which supports fast waste elimination.

There is a remedy that recommends drinking the juice of 4 lemons every day on an empty stomach for two weeks. However, I am not so sure about how effective this will be, so I prefer adding 4 tablespoons of lemon juice in a glass of warm water and drinking this on an empty stomach.

Peppermint

It is known that peppermint aids proper digestion since it stimulates bile flow as well as the rest of the digestive secretions. However, this fresh herb also helps in getting rid of gallbladder pain and relaxing the spasms.

Add a teaspoon of dried peppermint in a cup of boiled water. Strain after five minutes and enjoy the warm tea between meals.

Vegetable Juice

Make sure to drink vegetable juices on regular basis. If you don't own a juicer and have a gallstone, I suggest you consider buying one, since drinking vegetable juices regularly can help you promote gallbladder health and keep symptoms from happening. A good mix is a beet, carrot, and cucumber juice.

Dandelion

Dandelion is one of the most helpful ingredients when it comes to managing gallstones. It is packed with the compound called taraxacin that is known to support the excretion of bile from the liver. Besides that, dandelion is amazing at detoxifying the liver which is also important for preventing gallstone complications.

The best way to provide your body with the benefits of dandelion is to add about one tsp of dry dandelion root to a cup of hot water, and consuming it warm, after 5 minutes of steeping.

Milk Thistle

The substance silymarin found in milk thistle helps with bile production. You may be thinking that the more bile the higher the gallstone risk, however, that is the bile concentration. And producing more bile helps lower the bile concentration, which helps with flushing or dissolving gallstones when possible. Otherwise, the milk thistle will just make sure that the gallstones won't cause you any troubles.

Grind a teaspoon of milk thistle and combine it with three cups of water. Boil the mixture and let steep off heat for about 20 minutes. You can add some other herb or spice if you don't like the taste.

Castor Oil

Castor oil is packed with beneficial properties that can not only minimize the risk of gallstones but also reduce their number. It has antioxidant compounds that can reduce gallbladder pain and heal inflammation.

Warm a cup of cold pressed castor oil and soak a cloth in the oil, squeezing the excess. Place it on your stomach where your gallbladder is, and cover the cloth with a plastic wrap. Place a hot water bag on top of the wrap, and hold for 30 to 60 minutes. It is recommended to do this 2 or 3 times a week.

Pears

Pears are also great not only in reducing the symptoms from the pain caused by gallstones or other symptoms but also in preventing the gallstone's occurrence and growth. Its compound pectin will soften the cholesterol and make it easier for your body to flush it out.

Combine half a glass of pear juice with a half glass of hot water and drink the mixture. You can also peel and slice the pears, place them in a saucepan with water, cook them, and then eat and drink the compote.

*These natural remedies are not supposed to be used as a replacement or in addition to what your doctor has prescribed. Also, they do not replace a one-on-one consultation with your physician. Before you start taking any of these natural remedies, especially dandelion, milk thistle or peppermint, make sure to consult with your doctor, since some of them may interfere with some medical conditions or drug therapies.

The 6-Week Gallstone Diet Meal Plan

After days of research and multiple consultations with experts, I have created a 6-week meal plan for everyone who wants to manage their gallstones, reduce gallstone attacks and severe pain, minimize the risk of gallbladder lumps, prevent them from growing, and stop them from multiplying.

This meal plan is created carefully and meets the general standards of what a healthy and proper gallstone diet should be. However, know that every one of us is created differently, and so, our digestive system reacts differently to different foods. If you find some of the ingredients included in this meal plan to cause you discomfort or irritate your gallbladder, do not dismiss the whole meal plan as inaccurate. Instead, consult with your doctor and see the root of the problem. In many cases, the intolerance for certain foods may also be connected to another health problem. Then, simply replace the ingredient with something that your digestive tract can actually tolerate, and stick to leading a healthy, low-fat, and anti-inflammatory lifestyle that is free of gallstone attacks and severe abdominal pain.

If you thought that caring for you gallbladder and being careful not to trigger gallstone symptoms meant eating boring and flavorless food, then you couldn't be more wrong. This simple meal plan will give you a pretty good idea of how cooking for gallbladder health can be fun, healthy and irresistibly delicious.

WEEK 1

Day 1:

Breakfast:

1 slice of Whole Wheat Bread

1 tsp low-fat Butter

1 tbsp of Jam

1 Banana

A cup of Tea

Snack 1:

1 cup of low-fat Popcorn

1 glass of Apple and Carrot Juice

Lunch:

1 cup of Creamy Vegetable Soup

3 tbsp Whole-Grain Croutons

Caprese Salad

1 Peach

Snack 2:

½ cup Rice Pudding

3 Whole-Grain Biscuits

½ Apple

Dinner:

6 ounces Grilled Boneless and Skinless Chicken Breasts

¾ cup Mashed Potatoes

6 Asparagus Spears, steamed

½ Tomato

1 scoop of Healthy Banana Ice Cream (blended frozen Bananas)

Day 2:

Breakfast:

1 cup low-fat Oatmeal

½ cup Strawberry Slices

¼ cup Blueberries

A cup of Tea

1 cup of low-fat Chicken Stew

½ cup steamed Kale and Spinach Mix

¼ Zucchini, grilled

Snack 1:

1 Rice Cake

1 Whole-Grain and Sugar-Free Muffin

½ cup of Skim Milk

Day 3:

Breakfast:

1 English Muffin

Lunch:

½ Tomato

A Lean 3-ounce Beef Pattie

2 tbsp Cottage Cheese

1 Whole-Grain Bun

1 Banana

½ Tomato

A cup of Tea

A handful of Lettuce

A Veggie Juice

Snack 2:

Snack 1:

A handful of Almonds

2 tbsp Hummus

1 Pear

4 Baby Carrots

½ cup Blackberries

½ Pepper, sliced

1 tbsp Cream Cheese

Dinner:

6 Whole-Grain Crackers

Lunch:

1 cup of White Bean Soup

1 slice of Whole Grain Bread

½ cup of shredded Cabbage

1 Apricot

Snack 2:

¾ cup Fruit

2 tbsp Blueberries

1 tbsp seeds by choice

2 tbsp chopped Nuts by choice

1 Whole- Grain Cracker, crumbed

Dinner:

4-ounce Low-Fat Fish Fillet

½ cup cubed and steamed Sweet Potatoes

1 cup of Arugula, Cherry Tomato, and Pepper Salad

¾ cup Frozen Yogurt made with low-fat Yogurt and Fresh Fruits

Day 4:

Breakfast:

1 Whole-Grain Bagel

2 tablespoons low-fat Cream Cheese

2 Tomato Slices

1 ounce smoked Salmon

½ Grapefruit

A cup of Tea

Snack 1:

1 cup Melon Cubes

1 Handful of Hazelnuts

Lunch:

1 cup low-fat Chicken Soup

1 slice of Whole-Grain Loaf

½ cup of chopped and grilled Veggies

½ cup Blackberries

Snack 2:

1 cup of low-fat Popcorn

1 glass of Lemonade

1 Peach

Dinner:

½ cup steamed Peas

4-ounce grilled Turkey Breast, boneless and skinless

½ cup of mashed Potatoes

1 Carrot, steamed

1 cup Salad of mixed greens

1 small Apple

Day 5:

Breakfast:

1 Hardboiled Egg

2 slices of Whole Grain Bread, toasted

2 tsp low-fat Butter

1/2 Orange

1 glass of Apple Juice

Snack 1:

1 Bran Muffin

½ cup Skim Milk

½ Apple

Lunch:

1 cup low-fat Lentil Soup

1 ounce low-fat Cheese

1 cup mixed salad of greens, tomatoes, peppers, and corn

1/2 Banana

Snack 2:

2 Whole-Grain and Sugar-Free Cookies

1 Peach

2 Figs

Dinner:

3 ounces Shrimp

½ cup sliced and grilled Mushrooms

½ cup baked sweet potatoes

2 tbsp diced Tomatoes drizzled with some olive oil

½ cup Berry Mix

Day 6:

Breakfast:

1 cup Whole Grain Cereal

½ cup Skim Milk

1 Pear

1 tbsp Blueberries

A cup of Tea

Snack 1:

2 tbsp Goji Berries

A handful of mixed Nuts

½ cup Watermelon Chunks

Lunch:

2 ounces of Lean Roast Beef

4 Lettuce Leaves

½ Tomato

½ Cucumber

½ Whole-Grain Bun

1 Carrot

2 tbsp Dressing with low-fat Yogurt and herbs of choice

Snack 2:

½ Avocado

½ cup Skim Yogurt

1 small Apple

2 tbsp Sunflower Seeds

Dinner:

½ cup cooked Brown Rice

½ cup cooked Chicken Cubes

½ cup sautéed Veggies by choice

½ cup Cherry Tomatoes, sliced

2 scoops of healthy Ice Cream (frozen and blended Fruits)

Day 7:

Breakfast:

2 Egg Whites, scrambled

½ Bell Pepper, cooked

2 White Button Mushrooms, sliced and cooked

1 slice of Whole Grain Bread, toasted

½ Grapefruit

A cup of Tea

Snack 1:

1 cup of low-fat Crisps

1 cup of Cherries

Lunch:

1 cup low-fat creamy Split Pea Soup

1 slice of Whole Grain Bread

½ cup low-fat Yogurt

1 cup Salad with Greens, Corn, Tomatoes, and Peppers

1 Tangerine

Snack 2:

1 cup Carrot Sticks

2 tbsp Cream Cheese

½ Cucumber, cut into strips

2 Whole-Grain Crackers Dinner:

1 ½ cup Whole Wheat Pasta, cooked

1/3 cup of healthy Bolognese sauce made with 2 ounces ground lean Beef, garlic, herbs, and 1 diced Tomato

1 glass of Carrot, Apple, and Lemon Juice

WEEK 2

Day 1:

Breakfast:

2 Whole Wheat Pancakes

½ Banana, sliced

½ cup Strawberries, sliced

½ Grapefruit

A cup of Tea

Snack 1:

1 cup of Green Grapes

1 ounce of Cottage Cheese

½ cup Watermelon Chunks

Lunch:

¼ cup Garbanzo Beans

½ cup mixed Greens

1 Sweet Potato, boiled and cubed

½ Tomato

¼ Cucumber

½ cup steamed Broccoli

1 glass of Apple, Beet, and Orange Juice

Snack 2:

A handful of Pumpkin Seeds

2 Figs

½ cup skim Yogurt

1 small Peach

Dinner:

½ Zucchini, grilled

4 ounces cooked and shredded Chicken Meat

½ cup steamed Green Beans

4 Cherry Tomatoes

2 tbsp diced Avocado

1 glass of Berry Juice

Day 2:

Breakfast:

2 slices of Whole Wheat Bread, toasted

1 tbsp of low fat Ricotta Cheese

2 slices of lean Ham

Juice of 2 Oranges

Snack 1:

½ cup low fat Rice Pudding

1 Peach

½ glass of Pomegranate Juice

Lunch:

1 cup of low-fat Fish Soup

2 tbsp Whole-Grain Croutons

1 cup of Arugula, Baby Spinach and Kale salad drizzled with olive oil and apple cider vinegar

1 Pear

Snack 2:

1 cup baked Kale Chips

½ cup Pineapple Chunks

½ glass of Black Currant Juice

Dinner:

4 Artichoke Hearts, steamed

4-ounce low-fat Fish Fillet such as Cod, grilled

1 Sweet Potato, mashed

1 Apricot

Day 3:

Breakfast:

1 cup low-fat Oatmeal

1 tbsp chopped Almonds

1 tbsp Raisins

½ Grapefruit

A cup of Tea

½ cup Red Grapes

Snack 1:

1 cup low-fat Popcorn

1 Pear

1 glass of Kiwi, Lemon and Cucumber Juice

Lunch:

1 Whole Wheat Pita Bread

2 ounces cooked and shredded Turkey Meat

¼ Tomato, sliced

¼ Pepper, sliced

1 tbsp Cottage Cheese

1 tsp chopped Parsley

Snack 2:

2 Rice Cakes

1 Apricot

Dinner:

½ cup Corn

1 Carrot, steamed

½ cup Shrimp

½ cup Brown Rice, cooked

½ cup Cherry Tomatoes, halved

½ Banana

Day 4:

Breakfast:

1 slice of Whole Wheat Bread, toasted

2 Avocado Slices

1 Poached Egg

1 Orange

A cup of Tea

Snack 1:

4 Whole-Grain Biscuits

½ cup Skim Milk

½ Banana

Lunch:

1 cup Zoodles (Zucchini Noodles)

3 tbsp Pesto Sauce

1 glass of Pomegranate Juice

A handful of Sunflower Seeds

Snack 2:

1 cup of mixed Berries

½ cup Skim Yogurt

1 Rice Cake

Dinner:

1 cup of low-fat Bean Chili

1 cup of Salad with mixed Greens drizzled with olive oil and apple cider vinegar

½ Tomato

½ cup Blueberries

Day 5:

Breakfast:

1 slice of Whole Wheat Bread, toasted

1 tsp low-fat Butter

1 tbsp Strawberry Jam

½ Grapefruit

A handful of Almonds

A cup of Tea

Snack 1:

4 Crackers

1 tbsp Hummus

¼ Cucumber

1 Carrot

1 Pear

Lunch:

1 cup of Creamy Vegetable Soup

3 tbsp Whole Wheat Croutons

½ Avocado

1 Peach

1 tbsp Pumpkin Seeds

Snack 2:

½ cup Skim Yogurt

2 Biscuits, crumbed

1 tbsp Blueberries

3 tbsp Raspberries

2 tbsp chopped Hazelnuts

Dinner:

1 cup of Lentil Stew

½ cup Cherry Tomatoes

1 slice of Whole Wheat Loaf

1 cup Mixed Greens with Olive Oil and Apple Cider Vinegar

1 scoop of Healthy Banana Ice Cream

Day 6:

Breakfast:

1 slice of Whole Wheat Bread, toasted

1 tbsp low fat Cream Cheese

¼ cup sautéed Mushrooms

1 Orange

A cup of Tea

Snack 1:

1 Mango

4 Whole Grain Crackers

1 glass of Carrot, Apple, and Lemon Juice

Lunch:

2 ounces cooked Fish

½ cup boiled Potatoes

1 Carrot

½ slice of Whole Wheat Bread

4 Asparagus Spears

½ cup Green Grapes

1 glass of Lemonade

Snack 2:

1 Banana

A handful of Pistachios

1 Fig

Dinner:

1 ½ cup Whole Wheat Pasta

2 ounces of cooked and shredded Chicken Meat

¼ cup cooked Peas

2 tbsp low fat Cottage Cheese

¼ cup cooked Corn

½ cup steamed Broccoli

1 glass of Black Currant Juice

Day 7:

Breakfast:

2 Whole Wheat Pancakes

3 tbsp skim Yogurt

2 tbsp Raspberries

2 tbsp Blueberries

1 Orange

Snack 1:

2 tbsp Hummus

½ Bell Pepper, cut into strips

½ Cucumber, cut into Strips

4 Baby Carrots

1 Peach

Lunch:

4 ounces of cooked Turkey Meat

51

½ cup Brown Rice

1 cup of Mixed Green Salad

1 Tangerine

Snack 2:

A smoothie made with 1 Kiwi, a handful of Baby Spinach, ¼ Beet, 1 Lemon. And ½ Avocado

Dinner:

1 cup Bean Chili

1 /2 cup sliced and grilled Zucchini

½ Tomato

1 slice of Whole Wheat Bread

½ cup Cherries

WEEK 3

Day 1:

Breakfast:

1 Hardboiled Egg

1 slice of Whole Wheat Bread

1 tbsp Cream Cheese

2 Tomato Slices

1 glass of Orange Juice

Snack 1:

4 Whole Wheat Crackers

1 ounce Low-Fat Cheese

1 cup Veggie Juice

Lunch:

1 Whole Wheat Tortilla

2 ounces cooked ground Lean Beef

¼ Tomato

¼ cup Corn

2 tbsp Beans

2 Lettuce Leaves

1 Peach

Snack 2:

1 Meringue

1 Plum

1 Rice Cake

Dinner:

6-ounce roast Chicken

½ cup baked Potatoes

2 Artichoke Hearts, steamed

½ cup Beet Salad

1 small Apple

Day 2:

Breakfast:

1 cup Chia Pudding made with low-fat Milk and soaked overnight

4 Strawberries, sliced

1 tbsp chopped Cashews

A cup of Tea

Snack 1:

1 cup of Frozen Yogurt (skim fat and with fruit)

2 Whole Grain Biscuits

Lunch:

1 cup of low-fat Chicken Noodle Soup

1 slice of Whole Wheat Bread

1 cup Baby Spinach Salad with Olive Oil and Apple Cider Vinegar

1 Pear

Snack 2:

1 cup low-fat Crisps

1 cup Cherries

1 glass of Apple and Peach Juice

Dinner:

4-ounce Pistachio Crusted Salmon Fillet

4 Asparagus Spears

4 Cherry Tomatoes

½ cup Brown Rice

1 Tangerine

Day 3:

Breakfast:

A Breakfast Smoothie Bowl made with ½ Avocado, 1 Banana, A handful of Almonds, 1 tbsp Chia Seeds, a handful of Baby Spinach, ¼ cup Pineapple chunks and ½ cup skim Yogurt

Snack 1:

1 Whole Wheat Muffin

½ cup Mango Chunks

Lunch:

1 cup baked Sweet Potatoes

1 tbsp Cottage Cheese

1 Carrot

2 Artichoke Hearts

½ Tomato

1 cup Mixed Green Salad

1 cup Pomegranate Juice

Snack 2:

A handful of Dried Fruits

A handful of Walnuts

Dinner:

Whole Wheat Pizza with 3 slices of lean Ham, 3 slices of low-fat Cheese, 3 Tomato slices and a handful of Corn

½ cup Red Grapes

Day 4:

Breakfast:

2 scrambled Egg Whites

a handful of Spinach

1 tbsp Cottage Cheese

1 slice of Whole Wheat Bread, toasted

½ Grapefruit

Snack 1:

1 cup baked Beet Chips

1 Apple

Lunch:

1 cup cooked Brown Rice

½ cup steamed Broccoli Florets

2 ounces cooked and shredded Chicken Meat

1 tbsp Cream Cheese

Snack 2:

3 Whole Grain Biscuits

½ cup Skim Milk

1 Apricot

Dinner:

4-ounce Lean Beef Pot Roast

1 cup steamed Baby Veggies

½ cup Baby Spinach with olive oil and apple cider vinegar

½ cup washed Potatoes

1 Tangerine

Day 5:

Breakfast:

½ Whole Wheat Bagel

1 tbsp low fat Cream Cheese

2 ounces smoked Salmon

1 Orange

A cup of Tea

Snack 1:

1 cup roasted Chickpeas

1 Peach

Lunch:

Green Bean Salad made with ½ cup Green Beans, ½ cup Brown Rice, ½ cup mixed Greens, ½ cup halved Cherry Tomatoes, ½ cucumber and 2 tbsp low fat Dressing

Snack 2:

1 Whole Wheat Muffin

½ cup Skim Milk

1 Apricot

Dinner:

1 cup mixed Shellfish

1 cup steamed Veggies

½ cup mashed Potatoes

1 tbsp Cream Cheese

A glass of Apple Juice

Day 6:

Breakfast:

1 English Muffin

1 Banana

½ cup Skim Milk

½ cup Strawberries, sliced

A cup of Tea

Snack 1:

A handful of Cashews

2 Figs

Lunch:

A cup of low-fat creamy Vegetable Soup

3 tbsp Whole Wheat Croutons

1 tbsp Sunflower Seeds

1 cup of Lettuce , Tomato, Cucumber, and Pepper Salad with olive oil and Apple Cider Vinegar

1 Pear

Snack 2:

1 Hardboiled Egg

1 glass of Carrot, Lemon, and Apple Juice

Dinner:

1 cup low-fat Chicken Stew

1 slice of Whole Wheat Bread

1 cup mixed Green Salad

½ cup Pomegranate Molasses

Day 7:

Breakfast:

1 cup Whole Grain Cereals

½ cup Skim Milk

½ Banana

1 Orange

A cup of Tea

Snack 1:

1 cup of low-fat Popcorn

1 cup Pineapple Chunks

Lunch:

2 slices of Whole Wheat Bread

2 ounces of cooked Turkey Meat

2 Lettuce Leaves

1 tbsp Cream Cheese

2 Tomato Slices

1/4 Pepper, sliced

Snack 2:

1 cup Pretzels

1 tsp Mustard

1 Tangerine

Dinner:

1 cup cooked Okra

½ cup Cauliflower, steamed

1 tbsp Cream Cheese

4 ounces grilled Chicken

½ cup Beet Salad

½ cup Raspberries

WEEK 4

Day 1:

½ shredded Carrot

½ Avocado, mashed

1 slice of Whole Wheat Bread, toasted

1 poached Egg

¼ Tomato, sliced

½ Grapefruit

Snack 2:

8 Olives

4 Baby Carrots

½ Bell Pepper, cut into strips

2 tbsp Hummus

3 Whole Grain Crackers

Lunch:

1 cup Spaghetti Squash

¼ cup Tomato Sauce made from Fresh Tomatoes, Garlic, and Basil Leaves

1 Tangerine

Snack 1:

5 Whole Grain Biscuits

¼ cup Blueberries

½ cup skim Yogurt

Dinner:

4-ounce grilled Wild-Caught Fish Fillet

1 Sweet Potato, mashed

4 Artichoke Hearts

1 cup of Mixed Green Salad

A glass of Apple Juice

Day 2:

Breakfast:

1 cup Oatmeal

½ cup mixed Berries

A cup of Tea

Snack 1:

1 Cob of Corn

1 glass of Cucumber, Beet, and Apple Juice

Lunch:

1 cup of Clear Vegetable Soup

1 slice of Whole Wheat Bread

2 ounces of Fish

½ cup Green Beans

1 tbsp Cream Cheese

Snack 2:

3 Small Celery Sticks

4 Baby Carrots

½ Cucumber, cut into Strips

3 tbsp Hummus

Dinner:

1 Whole Wheat Bun

4 ounces of Turkey Pattie

2 Lettuce Leaves

1 tsp Mustard

2 Tomato Slices

1 glass of Minty Lemonade

Day 3:

Breakfast:

1 Whole Wheat Waffle

3 tbsp Skim Yogurt

½ Banana

2 tbsp Blueberries

1 Orange

Snack 1:

1 cup roasted Chickpeas

1 Tangerine

Lunch:

½ Avocado, mashed

½ cup Peas

4-ounces grilled Chicken

4 Cherry Tomatoes

1 Peach

Snack 2:

2 Rice Cakes

½ cup Skim Milk

4 Almonds

Dinner:

1 Bell Pepper stuffed with 2 tbsp cooked Brown Rice, 2 tbsp of chopped and sautéed Mushrooms, 1 tbsp Cream Cheese, and 2 tbsp mashed Beans

1 cup of Mixed Green Salad

½ cup Cherry Tomatoes halved

½ cup Blackberries

Day 4:

Breakfast:

1 slice of Whole Wheat Bread, toasted

1 tsp low-fat Butter

1 tbsp Fruit Jam

½ Banana

Snack 1:

4 Garlicky Jumbo Shrimp

1 Orange

Lunch:

¼ cup chopped Carrot

¼ cup Peas

¼ cup Corn

½ cup Green Beans

3 ounces shredded and cooked Turkey Meat

1 tbsp Dressing

½ cup Beet Salad

1 Apple

Snack 2:

A handful of Hazelnuts

½ cup Red Grapes

1 tbsp Goji Berries

Dinner:

3 ounces ground Lean Beef, cooked

1 Sweet Potato, baked

¼ Eggplant, roasted

1 cup of Lettuce, Tomato, and Carrot Salad

1 glass of Apple Juice

1 Pear

Day 5:

Breakfast:

1 cup cooked Quinoa

1 tbsp Blueberries

¼ Apple, grated

1 tbsp dried Apricots

5 Strawberries, sliced

2 tbsp skim Yogurt

½ Grapefruit

Snack 1:

1 Apple

4 Whole Grain Biscuits

½ cup Skim Milk

Lunch:

1 water canned Tuna

½ cup shredded Lettuce Leaves

A handful of Cherry Tomatoes

½ cup of Corn

½ Bell Pepper, sliced

½ Cucumber, sliced

1 Apricot

Snack 2:

1 cup Watermelon Chunks

1 ounce low-fat Cheese

Dinner:

4-ounce broiled Turkey Breast

1 cup Noodles

½ cup sautéed Mushrooms

½ cup shredded Cabbage with olive oil and lemon juice

½ cup Cherries

Day 6:

Breakfast:

Smoothie Bowl made with 2 tbsp Flaxseed, 1 Apple, a handful of Hazelnuts,

3 tbsp shredded Coconuts, Mango, a handful of Baby Spinach, Mint Leaves

Snack 1:

½ cup Frozen Red Grapes

1 cup Baked Carrot Chips

Lunch:

1 cup low-fat Minestrone Soup

1 slice of Whole Wheat Bread

4 Asparagus Spears

3 ounces cooked white Fish

½ Sweet Potato, boiled

Snack 2:

¾ cup Yogurt

½ cup Passion Fruit

1 tbsp chopped Nuts by choice

Dinner:

5 Turkey Meatballs

½ cup Mashed Potato

½ cup Peas

1 cup Salad of choice

½ cup Blueberries

A cup of Chickpea Soup

½ Whole Wheat Pita Bread

1 cup of Baby Spinach, Cherry Tomato, Carrot, and Cucumber Salad

1 Tangerine

Day 7:

Breakfast:

1 Hardboiled Egg

1 slice of Whole Wheat Bread, toasted

1 tsp low-fat Butter

2 slices of Lean Ham

½ Grapefruit

Snack 1:

A cob of Corn

A glass of Pomegranate Juice

Lunch:

Snack 2:

1 Whole Wheat Muffin

½ cup Skim Milk

Dinner:

1 cup Whole Wheat Pasta

4 ounces Chicken Meat, cubed and cooked

4 tbsp homemade Tomato Sauce

1 ounce low-fat Cheese of choice

1 Pear

WEEK 5

Day 1:

Breakfast:

1 Whole Wheat Savory Muffin

½ Avocado

½ cup skim Yogurt

1 Orange

Snack 2:

¾ cup Rice Pudding

1 glass of Blackberry Juice

Lunch:

½ Whole Wheat Bun

1 Veggie Pattie

1 tsp Mustard

1 ounce low-fat Cheese

Snack 2:

1 cup low-fat Popcorn

1 Pear

Dinner:

Stir fry made with 3 White Button Mushrooms, 4 ounces Chicken, a handful of Kale, ½ cup Broccoli, ¼ cup shredded Carrots

½ Tomato

1/2 cup Beet Salad

1 scoop Healthy Ice Cream

Day 2:

Breakfast:

2 Whole Wheat Pancakes

1 tbsp Cream Cheese

2 slices of Lean Ham

Juice of 2 Oranges

1 cup of Noodles

1 cup of steamed Veggies

1 cup of Mixed Greens Salad

1 glass of Pear and Lime Juice

Snack 1:

4 Crackers

1 Carrot, cut into strips

1 Cucumber, cut into strips

2 tbsp Hummus

Day 3:

Breakfast:

1 scrambled Egg

1 slice of Whole Wheat Bread, toasted

1 ounce of low-fat Cheese

Lunch:

Quinoa salad made with ½ cup Quinoa, ¼ cup Peas, ¼ cup Corn, A handful of Parsley,

¼ cup sautéed Mushrooms, 1 Tomato, 1 ounce Cream Cheese

¼ Tomato

1 Apple

A cup of Tea

Snack 2:

1 Banana

½ cup Skim Milk

2 Biscuits

Snack 1:

2 tbsp Guacamole

1 Bell Pepper, cut into strips

4 Crackers

Dinner:

1 cup of Shrimp

1 Peach

½ cup of Frozen Yogurt (low fat with fruits)

Lunch:

4 ounces Chicken Meat, cooked and shredded

½ cup Brown Rice

1 shredded Carrot

Caprese Salad

Snack 2:

A handful of Raisins

1 Apple

5 Almonds

Dinner:

1/2 Zucchini stuffed with 4 tbsp mashed Beans, 3 ounces lean ground meat, and 2 tbsp chopped sautéed mushrooms

1 cup Salad of choice

1 tbsp Cream Cheese

Day 4:

Breakfast:

1 slice of Whole Wheat Bread, toasted

1 tbsp Hummus

2 Avocado Slices

1 cup Red Grapes

Snack 1:

1 cup Pistachios

1 Tangerine

Lunch:

1 cup of Lentil Stew

½ Whole Wheat Pita Bread

½ cup of Mixed Greens with Olive Oil and Apple Cider Vinegar

Snack 2:

1 cup low-fat Popcorn

1/2 cup Pineapple Chunks

Dinner:

4-ounce Salmon or Cod fillet, grilled

½ cup Peas and Corns, mixed

1 Carrot

½ cup Mashed Potatoes

2 Artichoke Hearts

½ Tomatoes

A glass of Black Currant Juice

Day 5:

Breakfast:

½ Bagel

1 tsp low-fat Butter

1 tbsp Jam

½ Banana

A cup of Tea

Snack 1:

1 cup of baked Zucchini Chips

1 Peach

Lunch:

Potato Salad with 1 cup of cooked potato cubes, ½ cup Broccoli Florets, 3 tbsp Beans, 1 ounce cubed low-fat Feta Cheese, 1 chopped Carrot, and 1/2 Tomato

1 Orange

Snack 2:

½ cup skim Yogurt

2 tbsp Blueberries

1 tbsp Flaxseed

1 tbsp chopped Almonds

Dinner:

Whole Wheat Pizza topped with Zucchini, Eggplants, Tomatoes, Corn, Peppers, and 1 ounce low-fat Cheese

½ cup frozen Red Grapes

Day 6:

Breakfast:

1 cup cooked Millet

1 tbsp dried Fruit

1 tbsp chopped Nuts

¼ cup sliced Berries

A cup of Tea

Snack 1:

1 Whole Wheat Muffin

½ cup Skim Milk

½ Banana

Lunch:

4 ounces of cooked and shredded Fish

1 Sweet Potato, cooked and chopped

½ cup steamed Veggies

1 small Apple

Snack 2:

2 Rice Cakes

2 tbsp Goji Berries

1 Tangerine

Dinner:

1 cup of Bean Chili

1 slice of Whole Wheat Bread

½ cup Beet Salad

½ cup Cherry Tomatoes halved

1 Pear

Day 7:

Breakfast:

2 scrambled Egg Whites

1 ounce low-fat Cheese

½ Pretzel

½ cup skim Yogurt

1 Orange

Snack 1:

1 handful of Black Currants

4 Whole Grain Biscuits

½ Apple

Lunch:

1 cup of low-fat Chicken Noodle Soup

½ cup Brown Rice

¼ cup sautéed Mushrooms

½ Banana

Snack 2:

¾ cup Rice Pudding

1 Peach

Dinner:

4 Beef Meatballs

½ cup Mashed Potatoes

4 Steamed Asparagus Spears

½ cup Steamed Broccoli

1 cup of Mixed Green Salad

1 cup of Raspberries

WEEK 6

Day 1

Breakfast:

1 cup Oatmeal

2 tbsp Coconut Shavings

1 tbsp Dark Chocolate Shavings

1 Orange

Snack 1:

1 cup Pretzels

1 tsp Mustard

½ cup Cherries

Lunch:

1 Cob of Corn

4 ounces grilled Turkey Breast

1 cup of Salad by choice

2 tbsp diced Avocado

1 glass of Pear and Lime Juice

Snack 2:

2 tbsp Hummus

2 Celery Stalks

1 Carrot, cut into strips

½ cup Frozen Grapes

Dinner:

1 cup of Lean Beef Stew

½ Whole Wheat Pita Bread

¼ Grilled Zucchini with Garlic, Olive Oil, and Apple Cider Vinegar

½ cup of Blackberries

Day 2:

Breakfast:

2 slices of Whole Wheat Bread, toasted

2 tsp low-fat Butter

2 tbsp Sugar-Free Jam

Snack 2:

1 cup low-fat Popcorn

½ cup Mango Chunks

Lunch:

1 cup White Bean Soup

1 slice of Whole Wheat Bread

1 cup of Mixed Green Salad

½ Apple

Snack 2:

A handful of Almonds

2 Whole Grain Biscuits

½ cup Skim Milk

Dinner:

1 cup Whole Wheat Pasta

4 ounces cooked Chicken Meat

½ cup steamed Veggies

½ cup steamed Collard Greens, Kale, and Spinach

1 Peach

Day 3:

Breakfast:

2 Whole Wheat Pancakes

4 tbsp skim Yogurt

1/4 cup mashed Strawberries

Snack 1:

1 cup Pistachios

1 Homemade Fruit Popsicle

Lunch:

Fruit Salad with 1 Peach, 1 Apple, 1 Banana, 2 tbsp Blueberries, 2 tbsp dried Apricots, 1 tbsp Raisins, 2 tbsp chopped Almonds, 3 tbsp Skim Yogurt

Snack 2:

2 tbsp Hummus

4 Crackers

½ cup Beet Chips

Dinner:

2 Lobster Tails

¾ cup Brown Rice

½ cup Steamed Veggies

½ cup Cherry Tomatoes

1 glass of Lemonade

Day 4:

Breakfast:

½ Whole Wheat Bagel

1 tbsp Cream Cheese

2 ounces Smoked Salmon

5 Olives

A glass of Orange Juice

Snack 1:

2 Rice Cakes

1 Peach

Lunch:

1 Whole Wheat Tortilla

1 tbsp Pesto Sauce

2 ounces cooked and shredded Turkey Breast

¼ Pepper, sliced

¼ Tomato, sliced

1 Tangerine

Snack 2:

1 Banana

A handful of Hazelnuts

½ cup Skim Milk

Dinner:

A vegetable casserole with ¼ zucchini, ¼ bell pepper, ½ cup

Broccoli, 1 Tomato, ½ Turnip, ½ Potato, ½ cup Chickpeas, ½ Beans, 2 ounces low-fat cheese

A glass of Apple Juice

A tuna sandwich made with 2 slices of Whole Wheat Bread, 1 small water canned Tuna, 2 tsp low-fat mayonnaise, 2 lettuce leaves, and 2 tomato slices

Day 5:

Breakfast:

1 poached Egg

1 slice of Whole Wheat Bread, toasted

1 tbsp mashed Avocado with some lemon juice

2 Tomato Slices

1 Orange

Snack 1:

1 melon chunks

1 ounce Cottage Cheese

Lunch:

Snack 2:

½ cup skim Yogurt

½ cup Frozen Red Grapes

2 tbsp Blueberries

Dinner:

Whole Wheat Lasagna with homemade Bolognese sauce and low-fat cheese

1 glass of Lemonade

Day 6:

Breakfast:

1 cup Whole Grain Cereal

½ cup Milk

½ cup sliced Strawberries

Snack 1:

1 cup roasted Cauliflower

1 ounce Cream Cheese

4 Baby Carrots

Lunch:

1 cup clean Vegetable Soup

½ Whole Wheat Pita Bread

4 Jumbo Shrimp

½ cup Mixed Greens

1 Orange

Snack 2:

2 tbsp Goji Berries

1 Apple

5 Almonds

Dinner:

4 ounces lean Beef Pot Roast

½ cup baked Potatoes

½ cup steamed Veggies

½ cup Beet Salad

2 slices Garlic Bread (French loaf and made with low-fat butter)

1 glass of Pomegranate Juice

Day 7:

Breakfast:

1 Whole Wheat Waffle

1 tbsp Sugar-Free Jam

2 tbsp Blueberries

1 tsp low-fat Butter

1 glass of Orange Juice

Snack 1:

1 cup Roasted Chickpeas

1 Lemonade

Lunch:

4 ounces Cod

½ cup Brown Rice

½ cup Mixed Greens

1 Peach

2 tbsp Pesto Sauce

½ cup Blackberries

Snack 2:

½ cup skim Yogurt

1 tbsp Coconut Shavings

1 tbsp dried Apricots

1 tbsp Flaxseed

2 tbsp Black Currants

1 tbsp chopped Pistachios

Dinner:

1 cup Noodles

4 ounces cooked Chicken Meat

4 Artichoke Hearts

4 Asparagus Spears

½ cup Cherry Tomatoes

Dieting After Gallbladder Removal

If you want to avoid getting your gallbladder removed (and who doesn't) you should stick to the gallstone diet and general gallstone tips provided below. However, in some cases, removing the gallbladder is an inevitable thing. If that happens to you, don't despair. Living without a gallbladder may not be easy at first, but once you get to know your 'new' body you will see which foods are safe for you to eat, and which ones may cause you discomfort.

Because let's face it, the gallbladder is after all a digestive organ and even though it may not be essential, it still has some function that helps the flow of digestive fluids and aids proper digestion.

Once the gallbladder gets removed, bile will have no other choice but to flow from the liver directly to the small bowel. And while this is absolutely safe, the fact that there is no gallbladder present to collect and store the bile may cause diarrhea. Bile will no longer accumulate there, meaning that the quantities of secretions cannot be stored and broken down as they used to. But this is nothing serious. Limiting the fat intake and sticking to meals such as those in the meal plan from this book will ensure that you will have a healthy, painless and comfortable life even without a gallbladder.

Immediately after the surgery, the doctor will put you on a liquid diet. After you get your doctor's green light and it is safe for you to start introducing solids, here is what you should do in order to make things easier for your sensitive tummy, as well as your confused self:

77

- Introduce foods gradually. You may crave spaghetti Bolognese, but this is not the right meal for the days that follow the operation. Instead, choose steamed veggies, mashed potatoes, rice, and boiled chicken meat.

- Always choose the low-fat version as the low-fat is about to become your lifestyle.

- Have smaller portions after gallbladder removal. It is recommended to consume no more than 1,800 calories a day.

- Make sure your fat calories make up no more than 30 percent of your daily intake. For instance, if you are supposed to eat 1,800 calories a day on average, you shouldn't consume more than 60 grams of fat per day. One gram of fat contains 9 calories. 60 grams of fat means that we shouldn't consume more than 540 calories from fat a day (30% of 1800).

- Don't rush to get all of the high-fiber foods back in your diet. Make sure to leave the gas-producing foods for last. These include beans, seeds, nuts, broccoli, cabbage, cauliflower, brussel sprouts, etc.

- Keep track of your eating schedules and write down how you feel after meals. That will help you easily detect what causes you discomfort and what is safe for you to consume.

Now that you have the knowledge it takes for you to fight the gallstones, the next step is to simply create a shield in your gallbladder with your proper diet that will keep the gallstones from growing, moving, multiplying, or causing any discomfort.

Win a free

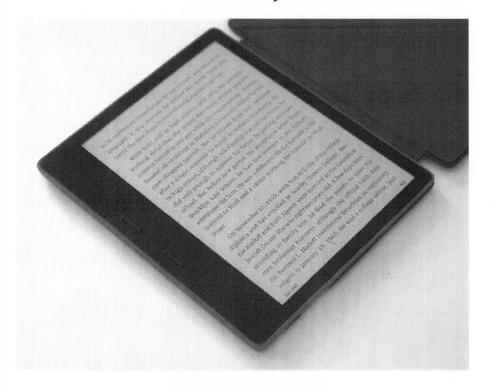

kindle
OASIS

[page intentionally left blank]

Made in United States
Orlando, FL
02 February 2022

14328519R00052